Cover Artwork by My Word!

Cover Photo by Mike Hirst

Back Cover Photo by Peter Turner

i

Succeed in Sport

- train - learn - adapt - improve -

Jackie Wilkinson

Paperback ISBN 1904312241
ISBN 13 - 9781904312246
Published in the UK and USA by MX Publishing
10, Kingfisher Close, Stansted Abbotts,
Hertfordshire, SG12 8LQ

This book is dedicated to

my late, and very great,

little Mum

FOREWORD

It gives me great pleasure to write the foreword for Jackie Wilkinson's book. I have known Jackie for many years and have been team-mates with her at both World and European Field Championships and have always admired her professionalism and passion for her sport.

I have been competing at an international level for over twenty years and have learned that it is essential to keep a training log to record your progress. This information is a powerful tool for development and for setting future goals. However, you don't want to spend valuable time writing copious notes or sitting at a computer screen entering data in order to complete complicated forms.

This book will appeal equally to both those people who are new to their chosen sport and those who have been doing what they've always done without having any clear goals or structure to their training. They will find it invaluable.

If you follow Jackie's sound and practical advice, you are sure to enjoy more focused practice sessions which will encourage you to achieve your full potential.

Alison Williamson
Olympic medallist, Archery

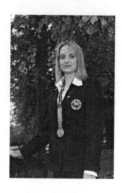

(Photo by Richard White)

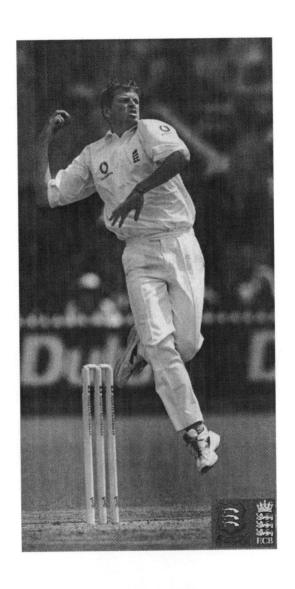

Peter Such - Cricket

England Team

ACKNOWLEDGEMENTS

As well as my own experience in archery, this book benefits from the sporting knowledge and expertise of the people named below. I would like to express my gratitude to everyone for their willingness to contribute. Including examples for many sports adds richness to the approach and clearly demonstrates how broadly it can be applied.

Hammer Throwing	Iain Holland, ex junior international hammer thrower.
Karate	David Christian, student of karate.
Running	Trevor Taylor, athlete and former secretary of Cumbria Athletics Association.
Badminton	Ian Graham, ex national junior badminton coach and manager.
Golf	Maurice Hirst, lifetime golfer.
Tennis	Sally Thompson, tennis player.
Curling	Terry Benest, amateur curler.

Many thanks to Alison Williamson, whose shooting I greatly admire, for her endorsement and for kindly writing the foreword. I also thank the following archers who have given their permission to be named: Jeff Pickett, Tom Bingham, Alan Wills, Jan Howells, Glyn Edwards.

I have appreciated the support and advice of Graham Stamford, Malcolm Cook, Iain Abernethy and my dear friend Noreen Price. Many others have offered ideas or contributed photographs. I valued the input of my Father, Maurice Hirst and Simon Degler who proof read the manuscript.

Roddie Grant of My Word! took on the important task of designing the cover and his wife, Janet was very patient with me when doing the figures. Gill Linder did the technique drawings and Wendy Selina lent her computing skills to help turn my cut and paste (literally) charts into electronic format.

My brother, Michael Hirst of Fireride, dealt with my technical needs and has made the charts available on the web-site he designed for me.

Thanks to Steve Emecz who showed his faith in this book by taking it on.

Finally and especially, thanks to my wonderful husband for allowing me to spend so many evenings writing.

ABOUT THE AUTHOR

5 times British Field Archery Champion, I have held several British records, competed at international level many times and enjoyed success at home and abroad. But it wasn't always this way.

At school, I was very poor at sport. My eyes don't point in the same direction, which means that they only work one at a time. This makes catching or hitting balls very difficult. I was frustrated by feeling sporty inside but not being able to do any of the games we played like netball, tennis and rounders. Then at university I discovered archery; a game of skill and coordination needing only one eye. As soon as I saw it, I wanted to have a go.

Early on I came last in most of the competitions I entered but I didn't care because I just loved doing it. Practising twice a week, I gradually improved. For the first few years I did target archery where everyone stands in a line indoors or outside on a field and shoots several dozen arrows at a line of targets. In 1984 I was working in Oxfordshire and my club took me to Wales to try field archery. The targets were set out on a steep, wooded hillside at various distances. We went round the course in groups of four as they do in golf. The club lent me some arrows; I lost two and bent all the rest; I was hooked!

Fortunately I have improved since those early days. When I started to win competitions, I began to take things more seriously. By getting advice from more experienced archers, I started to pay more attention to my equipment and fitness. Using video, I worked on my technique. My best results so far have been gold medals at the Circuit des 5 Nations in Luxembourg and Germany, a bronze (ladies team) at the European Championships, 8th place at the World Games and 10th place in the World Championships (sadly, field archery is not an Olympic sport) and I'm not finished yet.

My results have been helped by my interest in sports psychology and performance under pressure. Of course, keeping records using the charts described in this book, analysing the results and adapting my training, also helped me to succeed in sport.

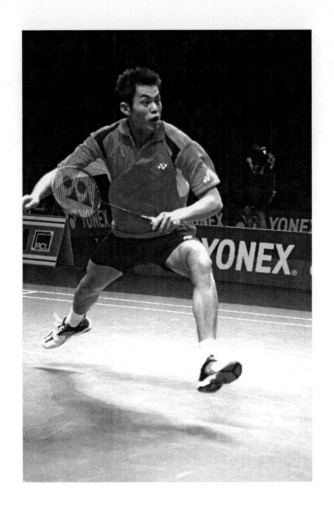

Lin Dan - Badminton

World No.1

(Photo By Peter Richardson)

CONTENTS

LIST OF FIGURES

CHAPTER 1

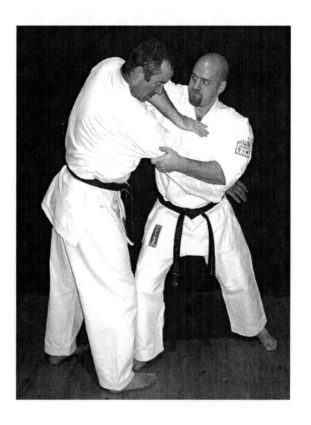

Iain Abernethy - Karate

5th Dan

INTRODUCTION

There is a man in our archery club who does sport purely for enjoyment. Jeff is a truly recreational archer with no desire to go to competitions, not even local friendly shoots. Sport provides an important space for him away from work and having been competitive before in another sport, he wants to avoid getting drawn back into the pressure of ever improving performance. He shoots with the club regularly and enjoys the relaxation of taking part. Tom on the other hand travels to many competitions around the area, but he doesn't go there to try and win. He goes for a change of scene, company and a nice day out.

There are plenty of Toms and Jeffs in the world of sport. They keep fit, get out, meet people and have lots of fun. That's great and I wish more people would do it, but this book is not for them. It is for those of us who want to improve, be the best we can, pit ourselves against others and win. Or, forsaking competition, those who strive for mastery of their art where the only competitor is yourself and the goal is to push the limits of what is possible and realise your full potential. Others with a spiritual faith, want to bring glory to God by using fully the gifts they have been given, in the way that Eric Liddell did with his running.

You can improve in anything; sport, your job, driving and so on, just by doing more of it, but at some point your performance will plateau. Unless you come up with a different approach, you won't progress any further. Here is a way of finding out how to keep improving.

The method I am going to share with you has come from my experience as a sports person competing in field archery at club, county, national and international level over the last 23 years. It is not a fancy theory and I do not claim to be an expert. I am just a competitive person who likes to do things well. It works for me and it will work for you, whatever your sport.

In 1991 I was selected to represent Great Britain at the Dutch Open in The Hague. Up to that time it didn't really matter when I shot well and when I shot badly. But there I was, at an event where I had to perform my best, TODAY. I began to wonder about the factors that affected me. How could I find out what helped and what hindered?

I had read an excellent book, *With Winning in Mind* by Lanny Bassham. He recommended keeping notes of training, performance and goals. In a page a day he recorded all sorts of things about what he did and what happened. I liked the idea but doubted I could keep up writing a page a day; it was too much. I also knew that even if I could make myself write so much, I'd never read it again. And with so many pages it would be difficult to recognise the patterns I wanted to discover.

I decided to find a more visual way of keeping a training diary. The chart I developed has a whole month on one page, where all the important data can be seen at a glance. Using this tool, I have continued to improve with 5 British Titles, a European team bronze and 10th place at the World Championships to my name (so far).

Currently, 32% of adults and 67% of young people in England participate regularly in sport with overall adult involvement at 46%.[1] That's millions of people doing sport. Of these many thousands are competitive. How many keep some sort of record of their training? Probably most. How many of those are able to use their notes to get quick, easy feedback to allow them to improve? Possibly very few.

If you are already performing at a high level in your sport, you may have sophisticated support available to you such as coaching, fitness testing, computer analysis and so on. The level at which high quality coaching support and performance feedback tools are available varies depending on your sport. For example, all this may be available at club level in track and field or swimming; for badminton it comes in at county level; for archery it is only for a few high level performers. For track runners there are clubs and coaches with

---

1   Sport England report Sports Equity Index for Regular Participation and Sports Participation and Ethnicity in England. www.sportengland.org.uk

training nights, structure and support. Many road runners are on their own. Even if you have sophisticated systems, you might still find simple charts like these useful; but until then, this method will be your main support for feedback, analysis and progression.

I have seen archers come to the club and shoot hour after hour, night after night, without getting any better at all. Others use their practice time well and enjoy success. Alan trains every day, shooting 100s of arrows a week and doing weights. He loves it and has the time to do it. He won a world championship gold with the men's team and is a lottery funded archer training for the Beijing Olympics. Jan has also represented Great Britain at international events many times, in spite of saying she doesn't practice much. Both have been British champions in their class. Jan spends much less time training than Alan; the important thing for them both is to use that time well.

Do you strive for excellence?

Do you push the limits of your ability?

Do you want to get the most back for what you put in?

Do you like to compete?

Do you want to win?

.....this book is for you.

Whether you are at club, county or national level, the tool I describe can help you.

You know what your own goals are. My purpose in writing this book is to give you a simple way to move nearer to achieving them. We'll look at finding the things that matter most for your sport, designing a chart to measure those things, using the results to modify your training programme and then planning the competition year.

I wish you every sporting success.

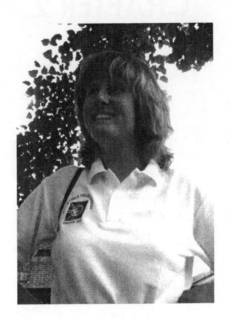

Jackie Wilkinson

(Photo by Peter Turner)

CHAPTER 2

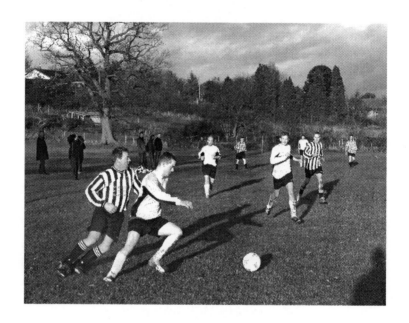

Football

(photo courtesy of Sportsreach)

THE LEARNING CYCLE

You love your sport. Having got past the novice stage, you're improving and want to get better and better. What do you need most? Feedback, that's what.

Many people have the physical capability to perform well. I watch them and wonder why they don't do better. The difference between the average club player and the international champion isn't so much to do with inherent physical characteristics; it's about using what they have to the fullest capacity.

We learn and adapt when we can see and interpret the results of our efforts. You will find this to be true if you try any new skill that has instantly visible results – throwing balls at a coconut shy perhaps. You can see if the ball goes high or low, left or right, and adjust pretty quickly. That's why they only give you three balls!

Feedback loops can be different lengths. Second by second, we continuously use the feedback from our eyes and sense of balance to walk straight and avoid bumping into people coming the other way.

If you have a coach, you will get prompt feedback on your technique, "your arm was higher that time." It is not easy to accurately translate what we feel into the actual positions of our limbs or the use of our muscles. You can watch videos of yourself to get objective evidence and find out whether you were doing what you thought.

In the longer term, keeping records of your practice and results can help you to refine your training plan so that you improve even more.   The next chapter looks at how to choose the things that contribute most to your sporting performance, and then we'll look at designing a chart to record them.   But before we dive in and look at the charts themselves, let's find out why this system works.

Learning is a cyclic process:

- Experience the experience
- Reflect and record
- Review and analyse
- Plan and prepare
- Experience the next experience
- And so on

Out of the four steps involved we all have a preference for that which we like to spend the most time on.   For the majority of sports people, the doing is what we love.   We have lots of experiences, good and bad, but may not be so good at reflecting on what happened and planning how to make it better next time. The best learning happens if we can manage to do all four parts, even just a little bit.

The charts I will show you are easy to use; it takes less than a minute after each event to capture everything you need, on a sheet you can carry in your kit bag.

Most coaches agree that it is important to keep records of training. There are many ways of doing this and some will appeal to you more than others. It is said that a picture is worth a thousand words. I used to write things down but then found that I never read them again. I wanted something that I could look at in a glance. I didn't want to do a page for every day because I knew that I would be overwhelmed by the sheer volume of information. I wanted to look at a picture which would tell me what the factors were that made me perform better or worse.

In this book, I present the method I developed for myself and have used for the last 15 years. I give examples from archery, badminton, hammer throwing, karate and running. Give it a try, adapting it to suit your own sport.

So as part of the learning cycle, it's good to reflect on what happened in your training session or tournament, but not until after you have finished. While you are out there, doing it, you need to be absorbed in the experience. You know the feeling; that wonderful connection. Mind and body in harmony; effortless movement, balance, coordination, decision making in the split second occurring at the subconscious level, equipment an extension of your own being. The Americans call it being in "the zone". It is also known as the flow state.

I have had days like this with my archery, tuning in to estimation of distances and angle of terrain, not thinking about my shooting, just doing it, pulling the bow and releasing the arrow smoothly, seeing it land in the centre of the target, coming in with a terrific score.

Most of all I've felt it when skiing. Turning left and right in fluid rhythm, in tune with the undulations of the snow, hearing the skis cut through the crisp surface - it's like flying.

Most of us have had a taste and it's what keeps us playing, training, and striving, wanting more. As Lanny Bassham says, "An outstanding performance is powerful. An outstanding performance is also easy." It is playing badly which is hard work.

So when you play your sport, play your sport; nothing else matters. Enjoy it. Then when you've finished, spend a minute or two to capture the learning.

Learn everything you can from coaches, others in your team or club and books on your sport. But most of all, learn from yourself. Get curious about what helps or hinders you. It's sometimes called, 'the difference that makes the difference'.

Personal excellence is a contest with yourself and there is much that you can learn from yourself if you will.

CHAPTER 3

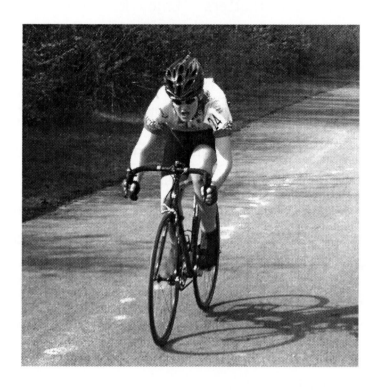

Simon Martindale - Cycling

SUCCESS FACTORS

Sporting performance can be broken down into the individual skills and strengths you need to put together for success. For archery I look at factors such as technique, arm strength, leg strength, flexibility, equipment set-up, ability to focus etc. They will be different for every sport.

Example success factors

Fitness:
    strength – stamina – speed – flexibility

Strength:
    legs – upper body – core strength

Skill:
    grip position – motion – balance

Mental:
    distraction control – focus – mood – confidence

Diet:
    during training - during competition - for
    avoidance of fatigue

Equipment:
    type – set up – maintenance – spares

Physical fitness and skill are obviously important. Other things may seem less so, but consider how they could affect you in the heat of competition.

My standard of equipment preparation changed dramatically after the inspiration of seeing a Frenchman competing in a medal finals match. As he shot his first arrow, something broke on his bow. He calmly swapped to his spare and put the other two arrows right beside the first, in the centre. I wanted to have his level of confidence that I could do the same.

Another of the major factors that separates the best from the rest is the mental aspect. It's easy to concentrate on physical training and forget that as you become more competitive, you need to be able to perform under pressure. The most important thing in golf is being able to visualise the shot. You need to be able to handle losing, and sometimes harder still, winning. Build mental toughness into your success factors and training. Use the chart to record the mental training you do and see what a difference it makes to your performance.

Clothing can be important too. Being soaked to the skin and freezing cold does little for your muscles or your mood. Archery is hardly ever called off for poor weather. I have shot in winds so strong I couldn't stand on my feet, horizontal rain, hail, snow, lightning and suffocating heat. It's best to sort out decent protection so that you can be as comfortable as possible.

Example success factors for a few sports

Curling	Hammer Throwing
<ul><li>Skill practice</li><li>Balance</li><li>Mental attitude</li><li>Tactical ability</li></ul>	<ul><li>Skill practice</li><li>Leg strength</li><li>Core strength</li></ul>
Badminton	**Karate**
<ul><li>Speed and agility</li><li>Aerobic capacity</li><li>Racket skills</li><li>Distraction control</li><li>Tactics</li></ul>	<ul><li>Skills practice</li><li>Aerobic fitness</li><li>Flexibility</li><li>Mental rehearsal of techniques</li><li>Mental toughness</li><li>Strength training</li></ul>
Archery	**Running**
<ul><li>Technique</li><li>Arm strength</li><li>Leg strength</li><li>Flexibility</li><li>Equipment</li><li>Ability to focus</li></ul>	<ul><li>Aerobic capacity</li><li>Miles run</li><li>Resting pulse rate</li><li>Diet</li><li>Posture and gait</li></ul>

If your sport is not included in the examples here, you can adapt the idea for yourself.

So the first thing is to identify your own success factors. Brainstorm[1] everything you can think of which might affect how well you play. Then look at the list again and reduce it down to what matters most. You will build your chart to include the training that you do to improve these key factors. For example, if aerobic capacity is a key factor for you, your chart should include aerobic training.

Know your own limits of information digestion and choose a number that you can sensibly manage. You might have thought of 76 factors but if you over-complicate your chart, you will come to resent filling it in and will find

---

1   Brainstorming is a way of generating lots of ideas. Just note down everything you can think of, even things that look daft (like how much you enjoyed an event). Do it as fast as you can. Don't worry at all whether ideas are good or bad at this stage – the aim is get as many as possible. It's more fun to do with a few friends. Once you cannot think of anything more, then you can start to judge what you have and throw things out. Sometimes the wacky ideas turn out to have some value so don't be surprised if you want to keep and use them.

it too cumbersome to analyse quickly. Later on you might want to increase the level of sophistication and start to break down your quality of execution into the individual components of your game.

Tennis: Attacking shots, defensive shots.
Or even broken down further: serve, forehand, backhand, lob, volley, smash.

Golf: Drive, second shot, chip, pitch, bunker shots, putt.

Hammer throwing: 3 turn and 4 turn throws (see the hammer throwing chart in the appendix for one way to record these separately).

Archery: Target, field, blank boss, elbow sling (I use hatched shading on the quantity section of the chart to denote elbow-sling work, which is a type of training).

Curling: Guard stones, draw, promote, strike.

Having decided the factors necessary to perform really well, think about your current level for each one. Compare this to what you would need to reach your personal sporting goal.

Don't compare yourself with some ultimate hypothetical level. I consider my flexibility to be good enough for archery even though I can't do the splits (a level of flexibility that only a gymnast really needs).

There is no need to compare yourself to other people. This is about you and your vision of what you want to achieve.

You can note your personal success factors here:

Enter specific factors under each category	Current level (out of 10)
Physical - - -	
Mental - - -	
Skills and techniques - - -	
Equipment and clothing - - -	
Diet / other - - -	

Plot the results in any way that pleases you. A table (Fig. 1) is fine or a bar chart (Fig. 3). I like to do mine on a circular diagram that looks like an archery target (Fig. 2). The important thing is to be able to identify the areas for improvement so that you can take action to bring those up to the level you want.

Rhythm	5
Equipment	9
Mental	7
Flexibility	10
Leg strength	9
Arm Strength	8

Figure 1 Performance profile presented as a table.

In this example, I'm only half way there for rhythm and need to do more work (skill gap of 5), but my flexibility is good enough already and just needs maintenance.

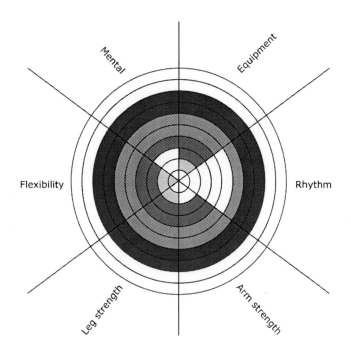

Figure 2
Performance profile presented as a target diagram

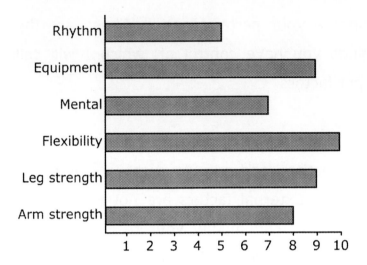

Figure 3
Performance profile presented as a bar chart

You are now developing an action plan by:

- identifying the key factors contributing to your success;
- objectively assessing your current performance;
- finding ways of strengthening your weaker areas.

The same factors that you choose for your performance profile will be used to create your personal record chart. This way you will be working on the right things to help you improve your performance. These are the things you have control of, which I will call input factors.

The chart will also include external factors, like weather, and outputs such as scores and results. External factors are not within your control but can modify your result. A good performance won't always produce a good result. Some of your training should be designed to minimise the effect of conditions, crowds, opponents etc.

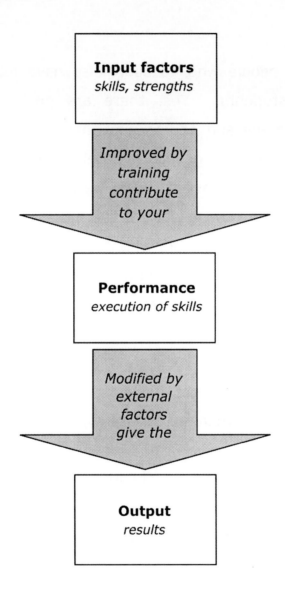

Figure 4

How a sporting result is created

Most people who do sport also have jobs or are students. Yes, there are professional footballers and golfers who make their living from and can devote all their time to their sport. They have the very best coaching and advice on how to stay at the top. There are even some amateurs who don't work and can do sport full-time, either by virtue of their personal circumstances, or through sponsorship.

For the rest of us, life is a juggling act. We can't train when we choose to, so we do what we can, when we can, fitted around study, work, looking after children and running a home. We train in the evenings (or notoriously for swimmers, very early in the mornings) and at weekends. Our time is precious so it is important to use it well. The charts will help you find the types and frequencies of training that suit you best.

CHAPTER 4

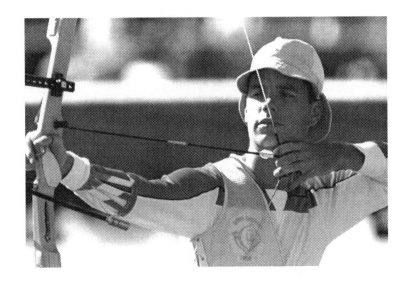

Jay Barrs - Archery

USA Olympic Gold Medalist, World Champion

(Photo – IOC/Olympic Museum Collections © CIO/F. Vanderlinde)

THE CHARTS

In the previous chapter, you identified the factors that contribute most to your sporting success. These are input factors, that is, the things which you bring to your sport and improve through your training. The next step is to construct your personal chart, which also needs to include any external factors that could affect the outcome and therefore result. We'll look at each of the following:

- quality
- quantity
- type of play
- other training
- external factors
- your results
- your overall placing in competitions

The design of your chart will depend on your sport. Make the key factors you have chosen easy to see. I have provided examples for archery, badminton, hammer throwing, karate and running. If you do one of these sports, you are welcome to use the example provided[1] but I expect you would still want to modify it in some way to suit you. Fig 5 shows a chart for archery. Charts for badminton, hammer throwing, karate and running are in the appendix.

I recommend one sheet for a month. If you like lots of detail you may want a sheet per week. If you train less often you might fit in all the information for a quarter. Do what you feel suits your style and training programme. It is easy to start with enthusiasm and do a lot at first but after a while it can become a

---

1   The charts are all available to download from my website if you want to use them as a starting point for your own design, in Open Office and Microsoft Excel formats. www.jackiewilkinson.co.uk

chore if you make it too complicated. The simpler you make the design, the easier it will be to carry on using it for months or years.

Make it visual. Once you have a few years' worth, you probably won't want to read it like War and Peace. I can lay my records out on the floor and see 5 years all in one go (see the photograph in the appendix). My best performances stand out and the training patterns that led to success are easy to identify.

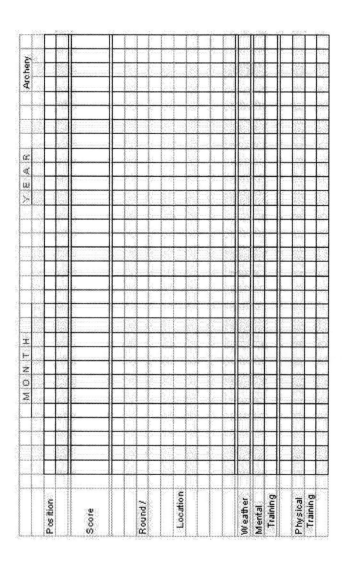

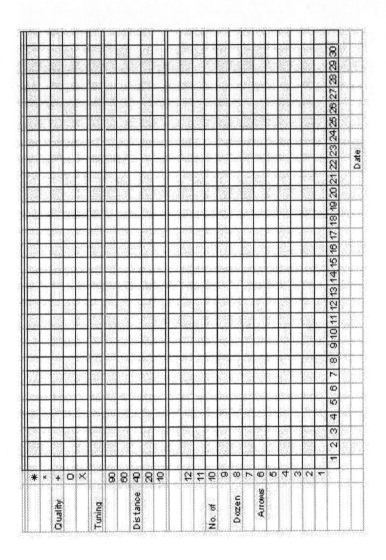

Figure 5

Example chart for archery

Quality

The most important thing to measure is quality of performance. This is the outcome you want to improve. Scores are often affected by weather or venue. Results depend on who else takes part. Quality of execution is all down to you. No one can control the quality of the track, the steepness of the course, the wind or their opponents. Concentrate on what you can control; your own performance. Improve that and scores and results will follow.

I measure quality based on how well I feel I executed the shots. The symbols shown below are how I denote the quality of my shooting. You will need to define your own levels of quality.

∗ This is the ultimate and is what we all hope for. These are the days when it flows. This is being 'in the zone'. Your focus is good, your decisions are right, the timing is on and you have rhythm. It's so easy you wonder why you ever find it hard. Most people who have played sport have experienced this feeling at some time and it's what keeps us coming back for more. The purpose of optimising your training is to have more of these high quality sessions.

* This is a day when it feels good but perhaps the result is not great or the flow is missing.

+ This is a day when you can do it but it's more effort and less effective. Some shots might be tense or sloppy. The rhythm might be off.

x This is a poor day when your body is out of alignment and every shot is a fight.

X This is a terrible day when you wish you hadn't bothered. It's hard work and nothing seems to go right whatever you do. Hopefully you won't have many of these.

Sometimes I will have a bad patch in the middle of a better day. I might put two symbols down together so that I know it was a mixture. 'Magic and Tragic' my friend Glyn calls it.

Occasionally, and frustratingly, the quality feels poor but my results are good. I still record this as poor on the quality scale.

Although there are those who want to win in any way and at any cost, most of the sports men and women I have spoken to agree that they consider their performance to be more important to them than the result. Playing well is satisfying even if another person does better. Playing badly but beating a competitor who has an injury or equipment problem is a hollow victory.

Quantity

Record the amount of your sport, both training and competition, that you do. I use the number of arrows shot. For running you could use distance covered and for karate, the time spent practising. Draw a bar graph at the bottom of the page. It's your measure of how much you do.

Type

Archery can be done inside, outside, on the flat, on slopes and at any distance from 5m to 180yds. I record the distance that I shoot. Divers might note the height of board they dived from. Hammer throwers will want to record the weight of hammer they threw and the number of turns. Badminton players can record matches and free-play. Runners might be on a track or the road, doing interval training, cross country or fell running. Sometimes I work on equipment set up, bow tuning and sight marks. I record this too.

Other training

In the early days I got better at archery just by doing more archery. Three years in, I met a teenager who was British junior champion. He talked with his coach about weight training and mental rehearsal. I thought it was a bit extreme (even having a coach was more than I was used to) but guess what I do now? Yes, weight training and mental rehearsal. In fact I use a range of other types of training to give me the strength, flexibility and stamina I need.

Someone once told me, 'fitness is the vehicle for your skill'. It won't make me shoot any individual arrow better but it will allow me to keep on shooting arrows well for 6 days of international competition.

If you have a job, as I do, or you are at school, your time for training could be limited and sometimes you will come home feeling too drained to do anything. Use your imagination when thinking about what constitutes training. Including different activities will allow you to fit in what you can, when you can. A walk here, a bit of strenuous digging in the garden there. Don't limit your thinking to major workout sessions. Running and swimming are good for aerobic capacity, but so is dancing, or you could pedal an exercise bike while you read or watch the TV. All of these contribute to your improvement so record them on your chart.

I haven't included anything to do with warm-ups on the charts. That's because warming up should always be part of your routine. You can include it on your technique master if you like (see chapter 6).

External Factors

In spite of good quality execution of skills by yourself, your results can be affected by other things: the ice conditions in curling, the lighting for badminton or the grip and uniformity of the circle for hammer throwing.

Weather affects archery in the same way as it does golf. My first attempt at recording weather using numbers wasn't great. When looking at the sheets, I had to read the numbers and that went against my aim of not reading much. Now I use the same symbols for weather as I do for quality of execution. The big star is reserved for days when there is no weather i.e. no rain, no wind, not too hot or too cold, no glare from the sun; perfect conditions. Even indoor venues can be too hot or cold or have poor lighting.

Team mates are a factor in many sports. However high your own skill level, a win depends on everyone working together to set up and pull off the plays.

For player/opponent sports like tennis and bowls, competitors and how well they play are very important. Also, the way you perceive your opponent can affect your level of confidence and you will need mental strength sometimes to beat a sporting star who everyone thinks is better than you. Aside from the mental aspects, competitors do not affect individual sports like archery or long jump because your own performance is not dependent in any way on theirs.

Crowd size and mood can vary. Our international badminton players got a shock when they played with raucous crowds abroad. In the UK, spectators are more dignified and considerate in their support and wait until the point is won before they cheer and shout. The umpires at Wimbledon ensure strict crowd control for tennis matches. In other countries and cultures, you cannot assume any similar respect for your concentration.

Even before your event starts, external factors could have made a difference. What was work like the week before? Have you been on holiday? Are you ill? Did you have to drive to get to your event or did someone else bring you? Although I try to plan to avoid it, there have been times when I have had to work flat out in the few days before a shoot and then drive hundreds of miles to the venue. My body and mind were not in the best shape to perform when I arrived. That is the hard reality of amateur sport.

Women need to be aware of the affect of their menstrual cycle on their ability to perform. It helps to know how you will feel, physically and mentally at the different stages as the affects can be significant. Check well in advance of international events and if necessary, shift your cycle so that you are on your best week for the competition.

Results

I deliberately put competition placings at the top (1st, 2nd, 3rd etc) so that I can see a line of 1s at the head of the page (well that's what I'm hoping for). You might use Win/Lose/Draw or symbols of sad and smiley faces to represent success and failure.

Underneath my placing, I put my score. If you race, this could be your time. If you jump, it could be the height or length of your best jump for the day. A cricketer could use batting score and a golfer the number of stokes for the round. Whatever it is, it should be an objective, measurable result. I also note down where I was and the type of event.

Key

On the back of the chart I have a key. This has proved useful because I have made changes over the years so I sometimes need to check what I meant at the time. I try to make each type of training about the same exertion per unit, so digging the garden for a couple of hours is about the same as a 30 minute swim. The key only takes up a third of the page leaving plenty of space for notes (we'll look next at the sort of detailed notes you might want to make).

Here is the key that I use for archery. There are example keys for badminton, hammer throwing, karate and running in the appendix. I leave it up to you to develop your own key.

Key for physical training
A   Aerobics
E   Exercise (weights, circuits)
F   Flexibility
Sw   Swimming
W   Walking
            (personally, I don't do running!)

Key for type
E   Equipment maintenance
T   Tuning
S   Sight marks
Sl   Slope practice

Key for weather
*   Perfect. No weather
*   Good. Comfortable temperature.
            No wind or rain.
+   OK. Some breeze or showers.
            Bright or dim.
O   Poor. Wind or rain. Hot or cold.
            Fog.
X   Dreadful. Heavy rain, wind or snow.
i   Indoors

Key for mental training
        Visualisation (default)
PA   Positive affirmations
R   Relaxation exercises

Summary

Check that you have covered all the things that you think will be important. Once you have your chart you are ready to start collecting information. Figure 6 shows a completed archery chart. Be prepared to change your design after a month or two as you confirm the importance of the factors you have chosen and discover what you are comfortable with. Later we'll look at how to use the charts to learn about the training that gives you the best results. I also deal with planning the whole competition year.

Next though I'll cover a couple of other aspects you might want to include: detailed notes and a technique master sheet.

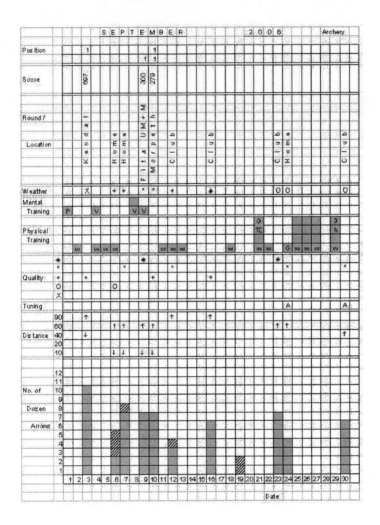

Figure 6

Completed chart for archery

57

CHAPTER 5

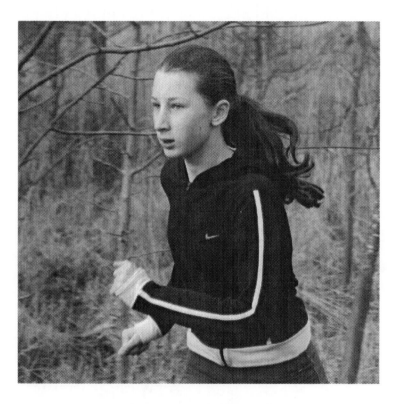

Rachel Hirst – Running

(Photo by Mike Hirst)

ADDING DETAILED NOTES

The whole basis of the charts is that you write very little. Having said that, it can be worth going a bit further sometimes.

On the back of the sheet underneath your key, there's lots of space to write notes. If you perform well, discover a technique point or have an idea, write it down. Going back over success is a form of reinforcement; it helps to breed future good performance. You probably know that you should speak in positives because what comes out of your mouth goes back in through your ears and your mind believes it. In the same way, what you write will sink into your mind via your eyes and through the acts of writing and remembering.

59

There is no need to write something every time you train. In a month, you might have 20 days with some form of activity and all of these should appear on your chart. In the same month, you might choose to make detailed notes only 2 or 3 times. The charts will still work without the notes but this extra detail can also be beneficial.

Example of detailed notes which I made at the European Championships.

Before trip
4th   Shooting well. Checked spare string. Group testing arrows.

Practice
11th   Number one bow, sight marks spot on at all distances. Mental training – circle of excellence. Visualisation. Made a small alteration to waterproof to tighten sleeve.

12th   Tried out waterproof (in the blazing sun). Fine.

Qualifying rounds

13th   Estimation mostly very good.   Started off shooting superbly.   Thunder, lightning, hail, heavy, cold rain.   Fingers got stiff and wouldn't let go smoothly. Glad of good waterproof.

14th   Shooting better. Good control. Timing within limit. Through cut to top 16.

Elimination round

15th   Physically and mentally strong.   Shot well but didn't make the cut to top 8.

Team event

16th   Scared to death; shook like a jelly. Weather cold and windy. Crowds and cameras. Shot superbly. Very pleased.

CHAPTER 6

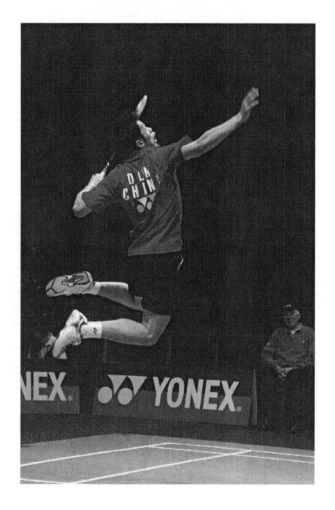

Lin Dan - Badminton

World No.1

(Photo By Peter Richardson)

TECHNIQUE MASTER PLAN

Separate from the record chart, I have a technique master plan. First of all, it covers the basics which make up my shot sequence including the placement of bow hand, breathing pattern and key words which I think of during the shot. Then it includes extra tips for specific circumstances such as shooting on slopes.

The technique master changes over the years as I learn new ways of making a better shot. So when I discovered that keeping my front shoulder low produced a stronger shot, I added a note. By collecting together in one place all the components, I have a complete description of the whole shot sequence which I can refer to. If I find a better way to do a particular part, I put it in and cross out the old notes. It evolves all the time.

I have not included warm ups in the example training record charts since warming up should be done every time you train or compete. The technique master is a good place where you can write down your warm-up routines. These will change and develop over the years and should including the best combination of physical, mental and spiritual preparation.

Example extract from archery technique master

General: Breathe in; raise bow. Set bow arm with shoulder low. Bow hand relaxed on grip. Align sight and string with target at pre-draw. Firm anchor. Aim. Stay strong right to follow-through.

Uphill: Move hips towards the hill. Set body angle and sight on target before drawing bow. Pull using back muscles. For extreme angle, stand with back to the target and swivel from the waist.

Downhill: Upper foot forwards with knee bent for stability. Let bow fall out of hand as the shot is made.

Diagrams are useful to remind you of body position and sequence of movement.

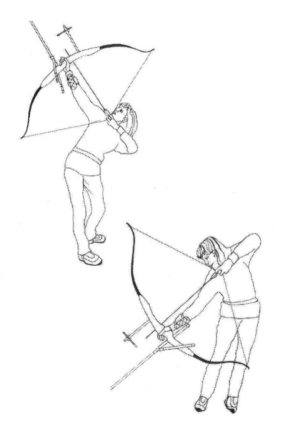

Figure 7

Body positions for shooting up and down.

Example extract from hammer throwing technique master

Warm up to include throws with a 1kg or 2kg hammer.

Dragging the hammer – watch hammer head during rotations, in particular when entering on first turn.

Standing up during turns due to loss of stability – focus on sitting down to squat position.

Under rotating – focus on fast right foot into 180^0 position square to shoulders.

Lack of hammer release – ensure plane of hammer increases during turns countered by increased squatting to final stand up release point.

I have a technique master for skiing too. I only ski once a year on holiday so this is useful to remind me of the key points.

Example extract from skiing technique master

Ski poles parallel to the skis.

Keep the line of the hands perpendicular to the skis to give sideways stability, like a tight-rope walker.

Raise for turn using knees only. Body stays at same angle. Chest to fall line.

Pivot from the little finger to plant the pole without lifting the arm.

Uphill ski slightly in front when traversing.

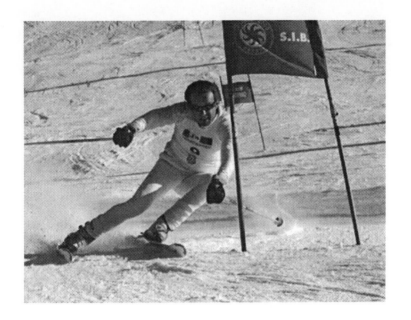

Alfredo Cantoni – Skiing

(Photo By Alberto Sosio)

CHAPTER 7

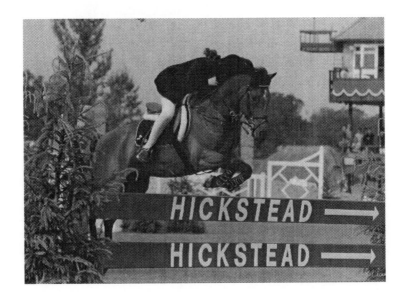

Joanna Harrison – Show Jumping

(Photo by Anthony Reynolds LMPA)

PATTERNS, CHANGES AND IMPROVEMENTS

Do you know whether you perform better the more you train? Does your performance continue to improve if your train more and more … and more? There will be a point when it becomes too much and you go past your peak and get worse instead of better. Do you know where that point is? For me the relationship between training and performance looks something like the curve shown below.

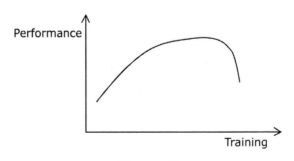

Figure 8
Training/performance curve

You have worked to collect all the information, now make it work for you.

Analyse your charts to find out what suits you best. Look for the stars meaning high quality of execution. I highlight the stars yellow so that they show up well. Quality performance of course ultimately leads to good results. Find out what you did when you had the most stars on the quality part of your sheet.

Look at how much training you did, how often you did it, which types you did. Did you get the most benefit from strength training, aerobic training or a mixture of the two? See how big an impact mental training had on your competition results. In the run-up to international events, I increase the amount of mental training I do and this allows me to produce my best performance under pressure.

Which are the trends that stand out the most? I realised very quickly that if I practised a little bit every day, my performance deteriorated. It's better for me to do more in each session but fewer sessions, with rests in between. Knowing this, I have redesigned my training programme and no longer feel guilty that I don't shoot every day. You will discover what works best for you. Coaches and books might recommend how often and how much to train but one size does not fit all; you are unique. Your personal training charts will give you clues as to what suits you best.

One of the benefits of keeping records is that, "what gets measured, gets done." If you have less training to record this week than you did last week, you will want to do more in future. Having said that, if you have lots of time, don't make the mistake of assuming that you will get better and better by doing more and more. Keep your records, analyse the results and learn what works.

Find out if including other types of training could help you perform in your sport. Be imaginative. Weights and circuits are great but there are other ways to get strong. T'ai Chi has improved my balance and control. Yoga is good for flexibility.

Thinking about the year as a whole, is it better for you to have a break or carry on training all the time? After the last competition of the season, I often feel so spent that I take a month off. One year, however I still felt good. I thought I would carry on without my break and get a head start for the following year. Instead of the better results I expected, I ended up stale and jaded with very mixed quality of performance when I started competing the following spring.

My month off not only rests my body but also recharges my enthusiasm, leaving me hungry to get back to shooting afterwards. Without it, my motivation flags. Now I make sure that I always have my yearly rest.

Learn from the trends, make changes to your training schedule and see what effects they have. Don't change too many things at once though, or you may get confused about what is giving you the improved results.

From a starting point of haphazard training squeezed into every available moment of your life, you can begin to develop a weekly training plan which fits around your personal life and gives you the performance benefits you need, efficiently.

It might look something like this:

Monday	Rest – no training
Tuesday	Club night
Wednesday	Weights+ mental rehearsal
Thursday	Rest
Friday	Aerobic
Saturday	Club session
Sunday	Competition

So now you have closed the learning loop. You have taken your experiences, reflected on them and recorded them on the charts, analysed them and used the feedback to decide what you will do differently. You are using your time more efficiently and working on the factors that will maximise your performance.

Your weekly plan won't stay the same all the time but will vary at different points in the year.

We will look next at planning your year as a whole.

CHAPTER 8

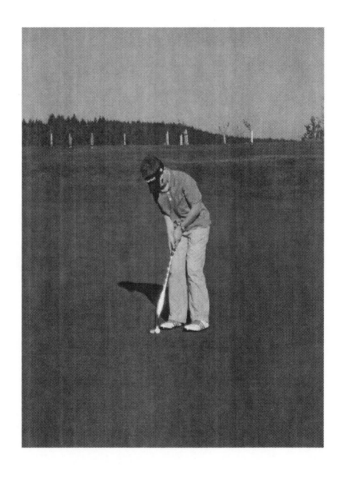

Matthew Wilkinson – Golf

(Photo by Paul Wilkinson)

PLANNING THE YEAR

By now you have set up a record chart including your own key success factors. Using what you have learned, you have understood how to adapt your training for improved performance. You can also use what you have discovered to plan your year.

Goals

When planning, start with your ultimate goal for the year. You know what that is. Perhaps you want to be the best in your club. You might aspire to make the county team or to represent your region. Or like Alan, you may want Olympic gold.

Work backwards from this goal, asking the question at each step, 'what would I have to do to achieve this?' The answers will generate mid and short term goals to work towards the ultimate goal. Then plan the training you will do to achieve those goals and monitor your progress towards them. Goals for each day can be related to your success factors and contribute to a particular physical attribute or skill element that you need to improve.

As part of your build up to a major event, plan to go to some smaller competitions to get you in the right mind-set. Think about how far you will have to travel and how long it will take to get there.

This example is an extract from the plan I drew up with the aim of becoming World Field Archery Champion. I haven't achieved my goal yet but the plan is valid and I will use it again next time.

Ultimate goal World Champion	Mid-term goal get selected for GB team	Short-term goals to have scores high enough
Finals rounds	Attend selection events	Perfect form (use video)
Qualifying rounds (likely score to make cut)	Book accommodation, time off work	Speed of shot
Practice at venue	Plan bow tuning to precede selection events	Practice sessions shooting 8 dozen minimum
Mental preparation	Other competition experience	Strength training - weights, stairs
Rest and relaxation	Positive affirmations	Aerobic training
2 bows fully tuned	Equipment checks and maintenance	Flexibility
Clothing and equipment suitable for conditions		Slope practice
Food and drink		Mental rehearsal

One year, I didn't check my arrows. Sitting by the window waiting to set off to the World Championships, I idly looked at a few. The fletchings were starting to come off! In a panic, I went through the rest. Nearly half of them needed attention and it was too late to redo them. Fortunately I have quite a lot of spares and usually I use the same three arrows for a whole week of competition. But I haven't been caught so ill prepared again.

General Planning

Looking at your record charts, you will see how often you were actually able to train (which may be rather less often than you planned or intended to). If you have a job, it isn't easy to fit in lots of training so your run-up to a big event will have to start earlier. Make allowances just in case there are times when you have to work late unexpectedly or a heavy day leaves you too tired to do anything but collapse in a comfy chair. Include in your planning enough time for equipment set up and maintenance. Put in duplicate sessions for any important activity so that if the weather is bad or you feel off colour, you still have another session allocated to get it done at another time. When thinking about what you want to do in the week ahead, recognise the realities of life and be prepared to be flexible.

The Year Plan

My competition season runs from March to October, with selection for the British team ending in May and big international events usually taking place in late summer. Any major changes in technique need to be done in the winter ready to be fully in place by the following spring.

If, like me, you know in advance when your major competitions will be, you can look at the overall pattern of preparation and training that gives you the best results. Before an international I like to build up my leg strength for about three weeks. The way I do it, that's enough time to get my legs strong enough to cope with demanding terrain for a week of competition. I don't need to be quite as strong for the rest of the year for normal two-day tournaments. I also increase the amount of mental training that I do and check all my equipment.

Weigh up whether it is better to go to an event every weekend or to be selective and choose only a few. Use your charts to find out what gives you your best performance.

Be careful with your run up. Start preparing too early and you risk going off the boil. Start too late and you won't be ready. It's a personal thing. No one can stay at their ultimate state of readiness all the time. You need to peak at the right moment.

Learn from your charts how long it takes you to bed-in a change of technique or get used to a new piece of equipment. By mapping out the dates of events that you will attend, you will know if there is enough time in between them to make any changes or if you will have to wait until the off-season. Having to compete when you are only half-way comfortable with something new is seriously bad news.

Rest

Remember that your commitment to rest and refresh yourself is as important as your commitment to train. Sports people can easily get carried away by their own enthusiasm and burn out or become susceptible to injury and illness. If you are tired you can push your body too far by training hard.

Rest needs to be built in throughout the week, between events and at key stages of the year. As I mentioned earlier, I take a big break after my last competition to refresh my body and mind before starting heavy winter training.

I live in the remote north of England and many of the events I need to attend are in the south of the country so I allow the whole of the previous day for the 7 or 8 hour drive and to recover from the journey.

Individual Competitions

Is it better for you to practice a lot well before a competition and then have a few days' rest?

Or do you develop more rhythm and consistency by continuing to practice right up to the start of the event?

Do you continue with physical training or have a break? Do you get better results under pressure if you increase the amount of mental training leading up to the event?

Do you find competition simulation useful, in your mental rehearsal at home and/or out on the practice field?

Your charts will help you to find the answers to these questions so that you can tailor your competition preparation specifically to bring the best out of yourself. When the pressure is on, knowing that you are ready will boost your confidence.

Finally

Now you have put it all together. This book may have helped you to think about training for your sport in a new way. You know the best types and frequencies of training for different point in the year. You can easily monitor your progress as your performance improves.

Using what you are learning from yourself, about yourself, you can move closer to your goals. I hope you reach them all.

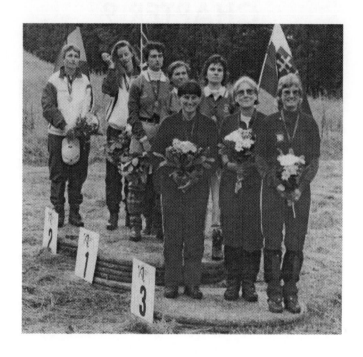

Great Britain ladies team winning bronze
at the European Championships
Ardesio, Italy, 1997

Left to right at the front,
Bev Taylor, Trish Lovell and Jackie Wilkinson

CHAPTER 9

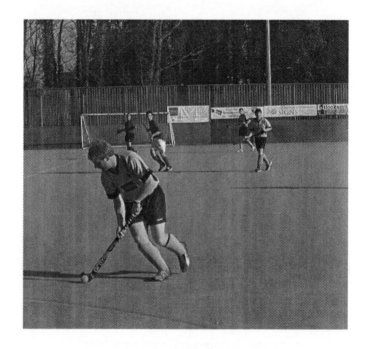

Hockey

(Photo by Sally Thompson)

FURTHER READING

I started by suggesting that sports people prefer doing sport to thinking about it. So I'm not going to say that you should do lots of reading but if you want to, here are some of my favourites.

Flexibility

Stretching, Bob Anderson, Pelham books, 1994
ISBN 0-7207-1351-X

Yoga for women, Nancy Phelan and Michael Volin, Arrow Books, 1981
ISBN 0 09 916990 8

Mental approach

With Winning in Mind, Lanny Bassham, X-Press, 1988
ISBN 0-9619194-2-6

In pursuit of Excellence, Terry Orlick, Leisure Press, 1990, ISBN 0-88011-380-4

The 7 Habits of Highly effective People, Steven R. Covey, Simon and Schuster Ltd, 1999, ISBN 0684858395

Ways of Learning

The Inner Game of Golf, Timothy Gallwey, Pan Books, 1986, ISBN 0-330-29512-8

Coaching for Performance, John Whitmore, Nicholas Brealey Publishing, 2002, ISBN 1-85788-303-9

Coaching pocketbook, Ian Fleming & Allan J.D. Taylor, Management Pocketbooks Ltd, 2003, ISBN 1-903776-19-8

Diet

Eat fat, get thin, Barry Groves, Vermilion, 2000, ISBN 0091825935

For more help finding the optimum diet for sport go to www.sense-uk.com

Archery Specific

Understanding Winning Archery, Al Henderson, Target Communications Corporation, 1983, ISBN 0-913305-00-6

The simple Art of Winning, Rick McKinney, Leo Planning, Inc, 1996

APPENDIX

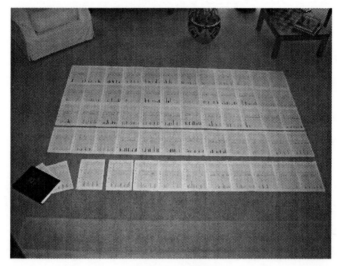

5 years' charts

EXAMPLE CHARTS

In this appendix are example charts, together with their keys, for badminton, hammer throwing, karate and running. The chart and key for archery are in chapter 3. Opposite is a photograph of 5 years' charts.

All of the charts are available to download from my website if you want to use them as a starting point for your own design, in Open Office and Microsoft Excel formats. www.jackiewilkinson.co.uk.

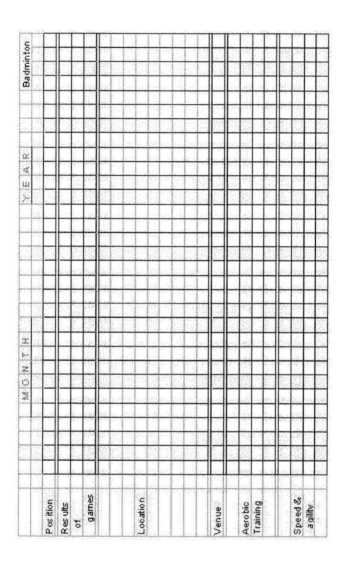

Chart for Badminton

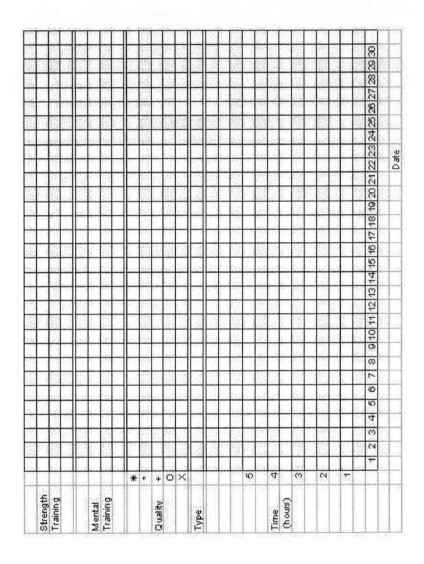

Badminton Key

Key for aerobic training

	On court (default)
	On court (default)
R	Running (one unit = X minutes)
C	Cycling
Sw	Swimming

Key for type of play
M	Matches
F	Free play
R	Racket skills
T	Tactical training

Key for mental training
V	Visualisation of skills
PA	Positive affirmations
R	Relaxation mental exercises

Key for venue
*	Perfect
*	Good. Comfortable temperature, good floor surface and lighting.
+	OK
0	Poor. Too hot or cold. Low ceiling. Bright background.
X	Dreadful

Appendix – Example Charts

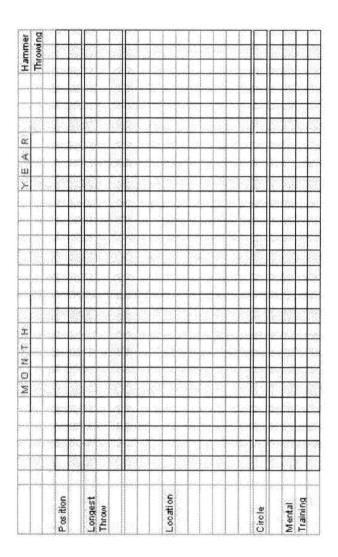

Chart for Hammer Throwing

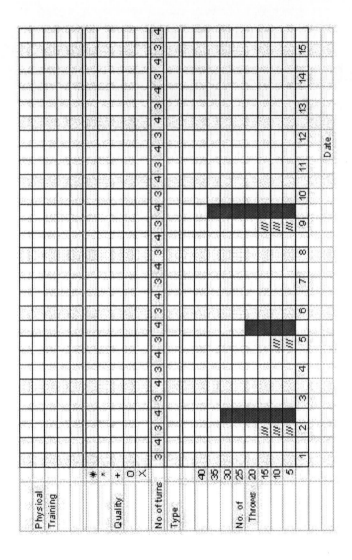

Hammer Throwing Key

Key for physical training

A   Aerobics, running, swimming
(one unit = X minutes)

W   Weight training, circuits, abs
(one unit = Y minutes)

F   Flexibility

Key for condition of hammer circle

✳   Perfect grip and uniformity.

*   Good.

+   OK. Some rough spots.

0   Poor. Wet, slippery.

X   Dreadful.

Key for mental training

V   Visualisation of throws

PA   Positive affirmations

R   Relaxation mental exercises

Key for type

         Standard 5kg hammer (default)

St   Straight hammer

H   Heavy

SH   Senior heavy

Appendix – Example Charts

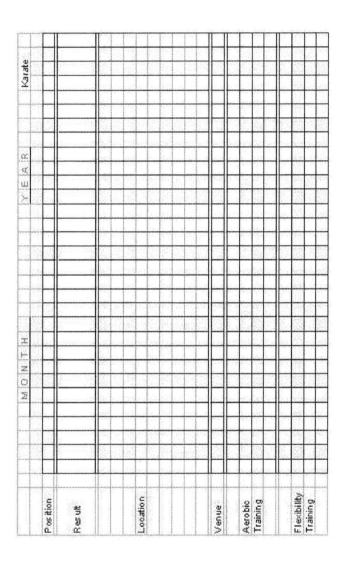

Chart for Karate

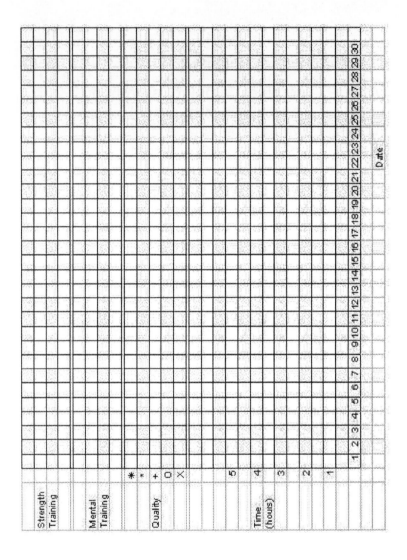

Karate Key

Key for physical training

A	Aerobics, running, swimming (one unit = X minutes)
W	Weight training, circuits, abs. (one unit = Y minutes)
F	Flexibility

Key for quality of venue

✱	Perfect floor surface, lighting and temperature.
*	Good.
+	OK. Some rough spots.
0	Poor.
X	Dreadful. Cold, dark, loose floor covering

Key for mental training

V	Visualisation of techniques
PA	Positive affirmations
R	Relaxation mental exercises

Appendix – Example Charts

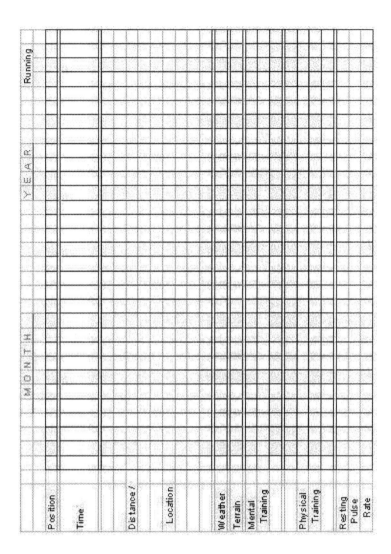

Chart for Running

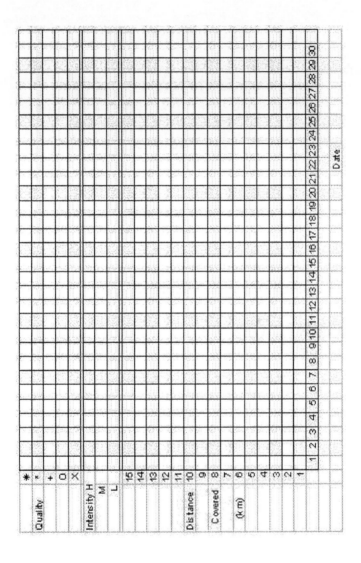

Running Key

Key for intensity
H	High eg. for 1/4 mile repetitions
M	Moderate eg. for 1 mile repetitions
L	Low eg. the level at which you can talk and continue over long distance

Key for other training
A	Aerobics swimming etc. (one unit = X minutes)
W	Weight training, circuits, abs etc. (one unit = Y minutes)
F	Flexibility, stretching

Key for mental training
V	Visualisation of running route
PA	Positive affirmations
R	Relaxation mental exercises

Key for weather
*	Perfect. No weather
*	Good. Comfortable temperature, light breeze.
+	OK. Some wind or showers.
0	Poor. Too hot or cold. Head wind.
X	Dreadful.

INDEX

Lightning Source UK Ltd.
Milton Keynes UK
09 November 2009

145998UK00001B/3/A